The Ketogenic Diet

A Century Old Diet that Works Effectively for Patients and Non-Patients Alike!

Disclaimer

What This eBook Tells You

The Ketogenic diet, which initially started off as a diet for pediatric epilepsy care, has now become one of the most trusted and fail-proof diets for patients and dieters alike. The reason is its lack of medicinal use and effectiveness. The best part about the Ketogenic diet, perhaps, is that it can be followed by children and adults alike. It is also not only limited for epilepsy patients but can also be used by people suffering from various other diseases.

This eBook will detail out all there is to know about the Ketogenic diet so that you can follow it in the best possible manner and acquire the results you seek. *The Ketogenic Diet* explains things like:

1. What the Ketogenic diet is, how it started, what are some common misconceptions about it and what its benefits are.
2. How the Ketogenic diet is suitable not only for those with epilepsy, but also for diabetes, Alzheimer and cancer patients.
3. Whether there are any side effects of the Ketogenic diet and who should follow it. Are you eligible for this diet?
4. Specific food items and exercises for this diet.
5. 30 recipes that range from breakfast to lunch, dinner to dessert and snacks too.

Hence, this book is a complete guide about what you need to do when following the Ketogenic diet. By the time you complete this book a lot of ideas will become clear to you and you will know just the right method to follow the Ketogenic diet program. So let us dive into a world of Ketogenic information!

Table of Contents

Introduction to the Ketogenic Diet

Throughout the centuries, many diets have come and gone. Some were prescribed by medical health professionals while others were only initiated by common people to gain their ideal weight and desired looks. These fad diets become popular because of their use by famous people, like celebrities, etc. There are very few diet programs that are developed keeping in mind some particular disease or ailment. The Ketogenic diet is one of them.

This eBook is written with the intent of making readers aware of the origins, reasons for, and benefits of this diet and whether it is suitable for you and if yes, then how you can follow it. Below is a short history of how the Ketogenic diet began, what changes it went through over the years and what shape it has become today. The only thing to remember is that following some things without change is a must, because this diet was constructed on certain key features and requirements. If you ignore them and try to modify them, you might not be able to achieve what you expected. Therefore, without further ado, let us understand the essence and practice of the Ketogenic diet.

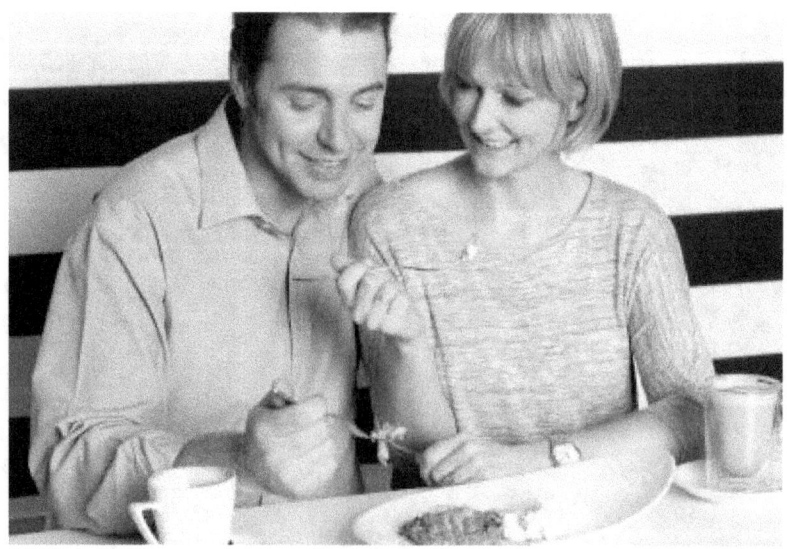

Travelling Back in Time to Understand the History

Before learning about what the Ketogenic diet actually is, there is a need to understand where and how it originated. What was the purpose behind the diet and is it really suitable for dieters? Can an average man, woman or child follow this diet, even though they might not be suffering from any medical condition? What are the repercussions? Will there be side effects? Benefits? If yes, then what? If no, then why didn't this diet become mainstream and commonly followed? Here are some answers for you.

How did the Ketogenic Diet Originate?

Originally developed in the early to mid-1900's, the Ketogenic diet was very famous during 1920's and 30's. However, research suggests that fasting, which is the core idea behind the Ketogenic diet, has been in practice since at least 500 BC. Of course it had not been fine tuned to be incorporated into a proper dietary system, but fasting was considered to be the main treatment for epilepsy and many other medical conditions. These facts come from a collection of ancient medical documents within the Hippocratic Corpus. One such piece in particular, in which the royal physician, Erasistratus, states that the only cure for epilepsy was a complete lack of food and drink. Later, with the arrival of Christianity, the King James Version of the Bible also mentions an incident where Jesus heals an epileptic boy through fasting and praying.

Fasting: A Precursor to the Ketogenic Diet

Proper research for the cure of epilepsy started in the early 1900's where medical health practitioners tried various methods, fasting and diets, medicines, and therapies to see what worked best. Fasting as a means of treatment can rightfully be called the precursor of the Ketogenic Diet. The first medical report of the effect of starvation among epileptic children was recorded by French doctors, Guelpa and Marie. In the United States, scientific research was also conducted on the effectiveness of fasting around the early 20th century.

Astoundingly, it was medical health guru, Bernarr Macfadden, who first brought fasting as a means of cure to the public eye. According to him, proper diet, exercise and regular fasting could not only keep an individual healthy; it could also cure many diseases like diabetes, asthma, epilepsy, eye problems, paralysis, impotence, bladder, liver and kidney diseases. These ideas were adopted by many medical health professionals, with Dr. H. Rawle Geyelin, an endocrinologist, among them.

Dr. Geyelin became the first medical doctor to report his theory to the American Medical Association and become acclaimed for it. Osteopathic physician, Hugh Conklin, also used this technique as a method for treating his patients. All patients, children and adults alike, were prescribed 18-25 days of fasting, where the patients were only allowed to drink water. Through this method, Conklin reported a 90% cure rate among kids and 50% cure rate among adults.

What is the Ketogenic Diet?

Conception and Progress

The concept of the Ketogenic diet actually came into existence in 1921, when two physicians Cobb and Lennox discovered that it was the presence ofacetone, acetic acid and betahydroxybutyric acid that occurred due to starvation, which caused the epilepsy to subside. The ketone bodies or ketonemia was produced by the liver due to the oxidation of particular fatty acids in the absence of carbohydrates.

A medical researcher at the Mayo Clinic, Dr. Russel Wilder determined that starvation or fasting was not the only way to produce these ketonemia in the body. According to him, with a low-carb, high-fat and a maintained protein diet, the body could work to produce the same level of ketone bodies in the blood.

Later, pediatrician Mynie Peterman formulated the original principles of the Ketogenic Diet, which contained a ratio of 1 gram of protein on 1 kg of body weight, only 10-15 grams of carbohydrates and the rest of the calories from fat. However, this diet was designed for children only and it showed highly positive results with 60% of the children recovering completely. The diet was also tried among adults showing positive results but was not as successful as was among children.

The diet was very popular for a decade, but with the advent of anticonvulsant drugs, its popularity dropped off and its use was mostly sidelined until the late 1990's.

The Actual Diet Program

As explained above, the Ketogenic diet ratios for patients and non-patients differs. For those with epilepsy and other medical ailments, the Ketogenic diet prescribes a daily dosage of a calorie intake divided among proteins, fats and carbohydrates. The ratio is 4:1 or 3:1 depending on dietary needs, with 4 grams of fat, 1 gram of protein and carbohydrates.

Most people children and adults alike, as well as those who tried the diet for weight loss who followed the Ketogenic diet reported that it leads to a leaner, healthier body and high energy levels.

The Ketogenic diet requires patients as well as ordinary dieters to cut down all foods that contain high levels of carbohydrates and instead focus on the intake of high fat food items. Research suggests that average dieter may lose as much as 6 pounds in the first 48 hours, which is comprised of the water weight a body has. An individual then progresses to lose ¼ to 2 pounds per day, depending on individualistic body differences.

In other words, the Ketogenic diet is a failsafe way of losing weight without any changes other than an alteration in what you eat.

Ketogenic Diet for Epilepsy

The Ketogenic diet started from fasting, which was practiced for many diseases, epilepsy the most common among them. As mentioned above, Hippocrates and his fellow physicians discovered in 500 BC that starvation was the best relief from epileptic seizures. Likewise, the Bible also claims the importance of fasting in epilepsy. Medical science proved in the early 1920's that with proper diet control and periods of abstinence from food and water could lead to complete recovery from epilepsy.

When the Ketogenic diet was formally initiated as a diet program, it was intended to be used for the purpose of epilepsy treatment among children. It was later modified to suit the requirements of adults as well and the outcome was positive in both instances. This shows that the Ketogenic Diet works wonderfully for the majority of people, especially children who follow it. Even if the diet does not cure epilepsy completely, it does lead to a reduction in seizures and a general good health overall.

When to Follow the Diet

The Ketogenic diets are mostly recommended to children or adults who do not respond to any type of medical treatments. This does not mean that you have to wait for the epileptic condition to worsen before starting the regimine. This diet seems to work best for patients suffering from Lennox-Gastaut syndrome.

Before starting the diet, it has to be kept in mind that exact amounts and instructions need to be followed. For example, the food has to be measured to the last gram before being consumed. Only then will optimum results be obtained. Also keep in mind that even though the Ketogenic diet works for most individuals, it may seem to have no effect on a small minority.

How to Follow it

In a typical Ketogenic diet, the calorie distribution is 4 grams of fats for every 1 gram of proteins and carbs. This means about 75-100 calories for 2.2 pounds of body weight and 2 grams of protein for every kg of body weight. The diet is started with a period of fasting which is then slowly eased into a prescribed amount of calorie and protein intake.

The diet can be continued for as short as 2 months or as long as two years of seizure control. In case of epilepsy, medication is continued along with the diet, to achieve the best results. Most studies highly recommend the use of Ketogenic diet in epilepsy as it is said to work for more than 60% of the patients. This is the reason why most hospitals continue to offer this program for epilepsy treatment.

Ketogenic Diet for Diabetes

Research suggests that the Ketogenic diet may also be beneficial in the control of type II diabetes. This is because the level of glucose in the blood is minimized to the point where it becomes almost zero. The reason why undertaking a Ketogenic diet is so effective for diabetes type II is that people first eat carbs and then control them with insulin injections. By following the Ketogenic diet, patients would be working on the root cause of the disease. They would not consume a high-glucose diet which would mean the blood sugar level will never increase. Hence there would be no cause for insulin stabilization. Research suggests that type 1 diabetes can also be treated with the Ketogenic diet but this needs to be discussed with a doctor first due to additional medical factors and in order to avoid any possible complications by undertaking without medical observation.

How the Ketogenic Diet Helps with Type II Diabetes

Diabetes II requires that the blood sugar be maintained at a lower level and remain stabilized. Likewise insulin should not fluctuate but remain reduced and stabilized. Controlling these two things reduces any risk of heart attack and organ damage. This is exactly what the Ketogenic diet does.

When following the Ketogenic diet, patients find it easier to:

1. Subtract foods that increase the chances of rising blood glucose. The Ketogenic diet requires the patient to reduce the intake of carbohydrates, which are the highest sources of sugar. Since most of the grain based foods are banned in the diet, this greatly helps in controlling the diabetic condition.
2. Since blood glucose level is maintained at a low level, chances of having a heart attack or metabolic diseases are drastically minimized.
3. Insulin resistance is also not developed when diabetic patients follow the Ketogenic diet. Symptoms of metabolic syndrome are also kept under tight controls.

Therefore, a diabetic patient who practices the Ketogenic diet will in time be able to bring the condition under complete control.

Ketogenic Diet for Cancer

The reason why the Ketogenic diet is prescribed for cancer is that cancerous cells need glucose to grow, but when they are deprived of that, they go into remission. This suggests that it is actually possible to starve your cancer! The basic idea is prevention instead of cure. Instead of trying to fight the cancer cells to make them disappear, the Ketogenic diet stops their growth by stopping their food supplies.

What the Ketogenic diet does is limit the amount of carbs consumed. Carbohydrates release glucose, which in turn is the primary growth source for cancerous cells. Since the carb resource is cut down, it is replaced by energy from fats. This means that your body remains healthy, but the cancer is slowly and gradually being killed off.

Even though not much research has been conducted on the effects of the Ketogenic diet on cancer patients, what little has been done clearly suggests that the diet is beneficial for most cancer patients, even those who have advanced conditions. There are little to no side effects and even if the diet does not reduce the size of the cancer, the diet will improve the conditions and quality of life.

KD Combined with Other Factors

Experts recommend that along with the Ketogenic diet (KD), cancer patients should add maximum sun exposure to their daily routine as Vitamin D in the sunlight reduces the reproduction and spreading of cancer cells throughout the body. Vitamin D also helps in regulating genetic expression and making the cancer cells differentiated.

Regular exercise is another must along with the diet. With the aid of exercise, cancer patients improve the circulation of immune cells as well as lower the insulin level in the blood. Proper sleep and controlled stress also aid in stopping the cancer from reproducing and growing in the body.

The above mentioned information shows that when cancer is treated with the Ketogenic diet, along with adequate sunlight exposure, regular exercise, plenty of sleep and reduced stress, the chances of recovery increase more than with medication alone.

Ketogenic Diet for Alzheimer's

Alzheimer's disease, the most commonly occurring form of dementia is a rising concern among European countries. As of yet, there is no cure for the disease. It is a degenerative disorder that worsens over time and ultimately leads to death. There are many medications that might slow the progressions of AD, but none have been able to cure it or improve general living conditions for patients.

New research suggests that the Ketogenic diet might actually work for patients suffering from Alzheimer's disease. Some studies show that the reason people develop Alzheimer's is because they have what is called 'neurofibrillary tangles' of protein in their brains, which develops as a resistance to rising insulin levels. Unlike type II diabetes, where resistance occurs in the liver, in AD this resistance occurs within the brain.

What does the Ketogenic Diet Do?

The Ketogenic diet works in the following manner:

1. The Ketogenic diet increases ketone bodies in blood, which results in a metabolized glucose level. This is because the ketone bodies are used as a primary energy source instead of glucose. The diet enforces the intake of a high fat, no carb diet which makes this process work.
2. Resistance and inflammation caused by insulin also do not take place, and this reduces the brain cells from any further damage.
3. Coconut oil is another item that is introduced in Alzheimer patients' diet. The oil contains medium chain fatty acids, which cannot stay in the body and therefore are immediately metabolized. What this does is produce extra ketone bodies in the blood stream allowing the brain to absorb energy that was reduced due to low glucose level.

Since there is still lack of research in this department, it can't be said with concrete surety that the Ketogenic diet will work well for all Alzheimer's patients. But evidence suggests that it can be helpful and will improve the quality of life for many patients.

Myths Surrounding the Ketogenic Diet

Like many other diet programs, there are many myths attached with the Ketogenic Diet as well. Below is a list of them, so that you can become aware that this diet is relatively risk-free and does not put you at risk if you follow it correctly:

Myth# 1: Ketogenic Diet is a Fad Diet

Many people believe that the Ketogenic diet is a fashionable diet that came into existence because of some media exposure. That is about as far from the truth as possible. As explained above, the diet has basically existed in essence before 500 BC and was gradually developed into what it is today through medical research and experimentation. A fad diet on the other hand is one that comes into fashion for some time and is forgotten in the wake of a new diet regime. This has not happened to the Ketogenic diet.

Myth# 2: KD Destroys Kidneys

The Ketogenic diet does not destroy kidneys because high protein diet does not harm the kidney, although it does increase the chances of developing a kidney stone. However, this issue can also be disregarded if you consume plenty of fluids to lower uric acid levels within the blood. People who are still resistant due to this slight possibility can take potassium citrate supplements as an extra precaution.

Myth# 3: Weight Loss Occurs because of Low Calorie Intake

It is true that KD reduces carb intake considerably, but this only shows that fat calories are the ones that can keep the body energetic and healthy by providing fuel. This proves that calories acquired from carbohydrates are not as necessary as once proclaimed. Rather, this only asserts the fact that a human body does need calories from carbs, but from a different source.

Myth# 4: Fast Weight Loss Occurs Which is Dangerous in the Long Run

Research suggests that a diet based on low carb intake is not only safer, but more sustaining than one which is dependent on fuel from carbs. This means that the Ketogenic diet not only helps with weight loss, it also improves the quality of life by making the body lean, strong and more energetic.

Myth# 5: Lack of Nutrients

The Ketogenic diet does not decrease the number of nutrients you consume, rather it increases them. The only thing it decreases is the level of sugar in your body, which instead of harming you, benefits the body greatly.

Myth# 6: The Ketogenic Diet is Dangerous

As far from the truth as possible! Some people are under the misconception that the Ketogenic diet leads to the production of ketoacidosis, which is produced when a person is suffering from type I diabetes and when the body is unable to regulate production of ketone bodies. This happens rarely and never occurs in a normal person, who is able to regulate sugar levels.

Myth# 7: High Fat Content Can Cause Heart Problems

Again, not true. This is because heart attacks are mostly caused by chronic inflammation.

Myth# 8: You Can't Exercise While on KD

This too is a false belief. It is true that the first three weeks of diet makes you relatively less prone to doing much exercise because your body is changing its fuel consumption from sugar to fat, which takes some time adjusting to. However, once your body has passed through the transition and is used to fat burning, you can easily exercise high intensity workout routines.

What Factors Make the Diet Successful?

The interesting thing to note is it has not been determined why the diet actually works in the first place. Research does give some pointers, but no absolute evidence has yet been determined. Different medical experts and researchers give different reasons for why this diet is so successful.

The Ketogenic Diet and Brain Functioning

What the Ketogenic diet does is increase the number of ketone bodies in the blood stream because of high fat intake. This means that instead of consuming energy from glucose, like the human body normally does, fuel comes from these ketones. Scientists suggest that these ketones are great as they increase the number of mitochondria, which provide energy to the brain. This boost in energy level might also be the reason that our brain becomes more alert, energetic and functions on a greater capacity. Neurons also become more powerful in resisting metabolic changes.

But that's not all. Another reason of the effectiveness of this diet is that because of an active and developed brain functioning, the body goes into a state of ketosis, where the levels of fat increase and carbohydrates decrease. The result is a rapidly working anti-inflammatory and antioxidant activity, which keeps neurons safe.

Lack of Carbs

The Ketogenic diet also works for so many people because it almost completely eliminates the intake of carbohydrates. This happens to be just the thing that many epileptics and cancer patients, as well as dieters need. Both in cases of epilepsy and cancer, the intake of glucose leads to a deteriorated condition. By removing carbs from the diets of these patients, what happens is that they are no longer susceptible to the factor that was helping increase their condition.

When it comes to obese people or ones who are trying to shed a few pounds, they also need to reduce the amount of sugars they consume. KD provides them the best health option possible. They don't lose energy, yet minus out the carbs from their diet.

Protein is Still There

Even though fat is the star of this diet and carbohydrate is reduced to the point where it becomes negligible, protein is still present within the diet. Keep in mind that you can never completely eliminate the intake of protein because it not only strengthens your muscles, bones and body organs after wear and tear; it also helps to improve your immune system. So never try to cut it out of your diet.

The percentage of protein is lessened to 15-20% in the Ketogenic diet. This means that you do get the required amount for body need but not enough to let amino acids be converted into glucose.

This way, the Ketogenic diet provides for all your nutritional needs, without storing up excess glucose released energy in the body. Lack of extra energy means you stay lean, fit and active without feeling any strains. Proteins and minerals are there to keep our muscles strong and your body energetic.

Some Other Factors

Some other factors that lead to the success of the Ketogenic diet include:

1. The state of ketosis results in a reduction of toxicity produced because of glutamate acid and which could lead to brain injury.
2. The Ketogenic diet increases amounts of inhibitory neurotransmitter or the GABA levels.
3. Cell death decreases when fuel is obtained from fats instead of carbohydrates.
4. Lack of carbs also reduces glutamate and oxidative stress.

Benefits of the Diet

When it comes to the benefits of the Ketogenic diet, there are many. Below is a whole list of them which will allow you to see whether or not this diet is the perfect one for your needs.

Fasting or Lack of Eating

Many research projects conducted over a long period of time show that fasting can lead to a cure from many diseases, from as basic as indigestion to as severe as epileptic seizures.

The Ketogenic diet works along similar ideology. The human body mostly gets its energy from glucose gained from carbohydrates. This form of energy is dangerous because it gets stored up in the body and is also the main feeding source for most diseases. Unlike the normal diet regime, the Ketogenic diet almost completely eliminates the intake of carbs and relies on the fuel gained from fats. This fuel is consumed as soon as it is released and is not stored up in the body. This state is known as ketosis. What this does is discourage the growth of many diseases and ailments.

In simple words, the Ketogenic diet keeps you fit and healthy without any excess carbs or dangerous accumulation of fat. Hence you remain fit and strong.

Better Metabolic System

The metabolic system remains strong and active when on the Ketogenic diet because it does not have to deal with the breakdown and absorption of glucose. Since there is a lack of sugar and grain consumption, the gut and other digestive organs remain stress-free.

Controlled Blood Pressure and Cholesterol

Again, since the amount of carb intake is less, blood pressure and cholesterol levels both remain in their perfect balanced states. Any arterial damage and inflammation also reduces and inflammatory chemicals would not be produced. The Ketogenic diet thus is not only great for diseases like epilepsy, but also works wonders for an overall better health condition.

Weight Loss

Even though you will consume more fats, the pounds will drop rapidly on the Ketogenic diet. Most of the weight gain occurs because of carbs and since they have been reduced significantly, weight is not just managed, it is reduced.

Another reason why weight loss occurs on this diet is the fast working metabolic system. All the energy is consumed and thereby you don't have any excess that can be stored as fat. But where does the energy go? It is used up by the mitochondria for all bodily functioning. And what little is left that is not used is excreted out of your body through urine.

One more reason for weight loss is that the Ketogenic diet produces an effect of satiety, which means that you don't get hunger pangs after a proper meal. The interesting thing to note is that this feeling continues for a long time, so much so that some dieters have reported that they forgot to take in a meal or two.

More Energy, Active Mind & Improved Mood

Most people, patients or not, report that when on the Ketogenic diet, they feel more active, highly alert and there is an elevation in their moods. This is again because of the energy released by fats that is essential for the growth and working of neurotransmitters. Essential fatty acids help the brain into functioning better than when it is provided with a carbs-based diet.

The ketone bodies produced due to this diet also help in stabilizing the neurotransmitters, dopamine and serotonin, which are responsible for mood and emotions. This way, you feel energetic and happier, keeping you in a positive mental state.

Peaceful Sleep

The Ketogenic diet cuts out sugary and grainy foods, which means that your digestive system does not have to go into an overdrive in order to complete absolute metabolism. What this heavy metabolic action does is make you lazy because your body is too busy with digestion and hence all other systems slow down. This means you end up sleeping at your desk every afternoon. This diet would allow a quicker metabolic activity leaving you feeling light and active. The end result is you get a full night's sleep and wake up fresh and happy.

Some researchers conclude that lack of grains and heavy sugar items also removes the chances of heartburn, which too leads to peaceful sleep.

Reduced Joint Pain

Many dieters stated that the Ketogenic diet led to reduced joint stiffness and pain. Reasons are yet unclear, but this can be very beneficial for those who have arthritis in their family background or are prone to the symptoms.

Ketogenic Diet for Weight Loss

Even though the Ketogenic diet is a medically researched and prescribed diet for many health conditions like epilepsy, Alzheimer's and diabetes, it has been gaining a lot of widespread popularity among the masses. The reason? Because it helps in losing weight fast! If you too want to adopt the Ketogenic diet program for weight loss, here is all the information you require:

Why the Weight Gain?

Before hitting you with scientific facts, get one thing very clear. Whether it is a few pounds you want to lose or dealing with obesity issues, the Ketogenic diet can work for both groups of people. So you can try it for about two months and see whether or not it works well for you. If it doesn't, you can always switch back.

Facts support the evidence that people who are following low-fat diets or routines, instead of losing fat, are gaining more. Statistics reveal that in the past three decades, since the conception and promotion of ideals that fats should be highly reduced, obesity and weight gain issues have increased three fold. This has worried many medical health researchers, who are now asserting the fact that fats are not harmful as long as they are taken from the right sources.

All of the above mentioned information depicts that it is not fats but rather carbohydrates that instigate weight gain and many illnesses like epilepsy, cancer, Alzheimer's and diabetes type II. Carbohydrates present in grains, sugar and processed foods as well trans-fats are the real culprits behind obesity.

How the Ketogenic Diet Plays a Role

What the Ketogenic diet does is it changes your routine diet drastically. The best part about the Ketogenic diet perhaps is that it provides with you all the nutrients and still helps you in shedding pounds. The reason for this is that the Ketogenic diet eliminates carbohydrates from the diet and increases the amount of fats consumed. The increase is such that the main fuel supply of the body switches from carbs to fat. Keep in mind though, that these fats are unprocessed fats which are easily burned and the ones not used are simply excreted in urine.

Medical health practitioners suggest that if you limit the intake of carbs to about 10-20 grams a day, weight loss will be rapid. But that's not all. You will grow stronger, leaner and feel more active throughout the day.

One of the most beneficial things about the Ketogenic diet is that not only will it work as a weight loss tool for you; it will also reduce your chances of developing high cholesterol, high blood pressure, heart diseases, stroke, diabetes and Alzheimer's. If you already have any of these conditions you will notice a significant reduction in the problems and will feel an overall energy boost.

When you consume high carbohydrate food, your body produces insulin to metabolize the glucose. But in the case of the Ketogenic diet, there is no insulin production since all the fuel is coming from fats which result in the production of ketone bodies. No insulin production means no inflammation and a reduction in the chances of acquiring diabetes, Alzheimer's and obesity.

Another reason why the diet helps you to lose weight is that when you are on a high fat diet, you tend to feel more satiated as the food gives you a feeling of fullness. This results in fewer hunger pangs and you tend to eat less. Your body also stops craving food because your blood glucose level is maintained.

The Requirements for the Ketogenic Diet

Many people feel that the Ketogenic diet can be hard to follow because it requires precision of the amount of food you consume every day. This might be true for individuals suffering from some illness, but if you want to go on the diet to achieve weight loss, there are some basic things you need to remember.

The first rule of the Ketogenic diet is that in a day you need to divide your food ratio to 70% fat, 20% protein and 10% carbohydrates. Also remember that increasing the amount of protein is not important for the body and would lead to a breakdown of the Ketogenic diet.

The second rule is that there are some foods and drinks you will have to drop completely. This is because they contain nothing but sugar and trans-fats, the exact opposite of what the Ketogenic diet promotes. These food/drink items include processed and packaged foods, fast foods and fizzy drinks.

And that is about it. These two rules can help you change the way you look, you feel and your body will be lean and strong without any nutritional deficit. This is great news for food lovers too, as they can eat all the fat they want, as long as it has nothing to do with trans-fats. By going on the Ketogenic diet, you will be able to enjoy meats and cooking in oil without having to worry about heart attacks or rising cholesterol.

Those people who are worried about their fiber intake due to lack of grains, can always consume non-starchy vegetables like Brussels sprouts and broccoli that are low in carbs but have high antioxidant properties and high fiber content. This way you can stay away from grains yet still stock up on your fiber needs.

Are there Any Side Effects to It?

Like with most other diet programs, the Ketogenic diet also has some side effects. The difference is that most of them aren't life threatening and can be overcome with care. Research also suggests that not everyone who followed the diet had to go through side effects, rather some experienced them more than others. Complications included:

1. Dehydration
2. Nausea
3. Dizziness, weakness, fatigue
4. Headache
5. Constipation
6. Kidney stone
7. Metabolic acidosis

The reason why dieters went through these side effects was because either they started by fasting or because their bodies took some time getting used to the problems. Research suggests that with adequate care and some supplements, these complications can easily be controlled. There is little to no evidence that suggests there may be any life threatening side effect that could severely deteriorate the condition of a dieter.

Even the more complex issue of suffering from a kidney stone took place only among 1 in 20 dieters. This too can be reduced by adding some proper food into the diet. Medical health practitioners advised that the Ketogenic diet is relatively risk free for both adults and children. Studies conducted on the long-term use of the Ketogenic diet for obesity also showed that there were no adverse side effects and its use over a long period of time is safe.

This shows that compared to any other fad diet, the Ketogenic diet is safe, effective, healthy and can be followed by patients and non-patients alike without any fear of harsh side effects.

Why Choose the Ketogenic Diet?

Enough evidence has been given above to show that the Ketogenic diet is relatively risk free and very effective. There are also some side effects of the Ketogenic diet, yet many people still tend to choose it and in recent times there has been a rise in its popularity. Perhaps one of the biggest reasons for this is that a lot of studies have been conducted on the diet and many people who have lost more than 100 pounds have come forward as witness to its functionality and efficacy.

But why should you choose it? If you have any disease like epilepsy, diabetes type II, heart issues, Alzheimer's or weight issues, then the chances of KD working for you are greater. Even if you are among that group of people who want to lose weight and then keep it that way, the Ketogenic diet is perfect for you. This is because it provides all the nutrients your body needs for a healthy outcome and does so without increasing any ailments or digestive issues.

If you fall among the group of people who are eligible for this diet, then without further thought, plunge into it. Speak to your doctor right away and get started! All you would need to do is try it for two months and decide whether or not it's working for you. The great thing is that even if does not show your desired results, you will come to no harm. Since all the foods and drinks used in the diet are completely natural, there is no chance of any damage.

The best way to find out if the diet works for you? Start following the Ketogenic diet and find out!

Can You Follow This Diet?

If you don't have diabetes type I and are not allergic to fat, then you are eligible for participating in the Ketogenic diet. A vast majority of people can follow this diet because there are little to no side effects, and the few complications that do exist, can be taken care of and easily remedied. Even though there is yet not enough research, studies are being conducted on how even diabetes type I can be treated with this diet with reduced risk of complications.

If you want to get over your obesity struggles or want to shed those pesky pounds, then the Ketogenic diet is perfect for you. Why? Because it works well for both of these problems! The reason this happens is because the biggest cause for obesity is too much carbohydrate consumption. The Ketogenic diet brings down average carbohydrate intake from 70-80% to only 10% a day.

When you follow this diet, you will be required to up the amount of fats you eat each day. Yes we have been ingrained to believe that fats are bad for your health, but that is only true for trans-fats because they get stored in the body and block arteries, thereby causing strokes and heart attacks. The good fats, also known as unsaturated fats, are the ones that can help you lose weight instead of gaining any. Research also suggests that by consuming more good fats instead of carbohydrates, you have a more likely chance of shedding those extra pounds.

When you consume these good fats in a higher dosage, your body metabolizes them and starts using them as the main source for energy instead of burning carbohydrates to produce glucose. Of course, proteins are also present in this diet, which means that any wear or tear of muscles or any other body part is kept upgraded.

This shows that almost everyone can follow the Ketogenic diet as it is does not lead to any disease or physical problem. Instead it is more likely to solve many of your existing ailments like indigestion, sleep apnea, heartburn, obesity, heart-related issues, hypertension and many others.

Cyclical Ketogenic Diet & Menu

The basic ideology of both the original Ketogenic diet and cyclical Ketogenic diet is the same. Both emphasize the reduction of carbohydrates which is to be replaced by high fat intake so that the body can function more efficiently.

Difference between the Ketogenic and Cyclical Ketogenic Diets

One major difference between both is that CKD has been designed specifically for body builders or those who are trying to lose weight and increase their muscle mass. In other words, cyclical Ketogenic diet is for those who want to develop muscle power that is suitable for high intensity activities like sports.

While the Ketogenic diet can be followed by everyone who wants to lose weight or has some particular illness like epilepsy, cancer, diabetes type II, etc., cyclical Ketogenic diet is for those who also want to work on their muscles, particularly body builders and athletes. Therefore, if you come under the list of people who are more interested in toning your body and developing muscles, cyclical Ketogenic diet is the one for you.

Another major difference between the two types of Ketogenic diets is that, in the cyclical Ketogenic diet there are periods where the dieters are required to consume high amounts of carbohydrates. This is because muscle glycogen, which is obtained from carbs, is the main source of energy for anaerobic exercise. What this does is it allows you to perform lifts and do other extensive exercises. Since these are essential for muscle building, you do need carbohydrates even though the first rule of the Ketogenic diet is lack of carbohydrate.

Managing Cyclical Ketogenic Diet

A simple rule of thumb and the easiest way to follow the cyclical Ketogenic diet is to follow the regular Ketogenic diet on all the weekdays and go crazy with carbs consumption on weekends. Of course, going crazy in limits is the key. You can eat any food you like, but bear in mind that you cannot overdo it for two reasons.

One; if you overdo the carbohydrate consumption, your body will store all the excess energy, which will ultimately lead to rapid weight gain instead of loss. It is best to not travel that road as not only will you lose motivation, it will be difficult starting all over again.

Two; if you consume too many carbs and sugars over the weekend, your body will find it difficult to control temptation and the food craving will resume, leading to more possible binge eating of undesirable foods. Do consume carbs, but make sure you don't overdo it. You don't want to give up in the middle of the muscle building program, do you?

But yes, unlike the original Ketogenic diet, you do get freedom where you can literally eat anything and everything your heart desires on break days. So enjoy them and build up some glycogen in your muscles for the extraneous exercise your muscles will need.

Exercises for the Ketogenic Diet

Most research suggests that people do not need to exercise when they are on the Ketogenic diet because weight loss naturally occurs, irrespective of whether or not you move your body. What needs to be kept in mind though is that exercise is not only important for weight loss and maintenance, but also for a healthy and active being. So whichever diet program you follow, be sure to continuously mix it with a particular workout program that best suits your needs and abilities.

Below are some exercise routines for both types of Ketogenic diet plans and you can follow whichever plan you have been following. Just make sure you don't overdo it on the exercise. Start slow and then increase both, number of minutes as well as intensity of the workout routine. Here are some exercises for you:

Exercise Routines for the Ketogenic Diet

Exercise is essential, whether you are on some kind of diet or not. This is because exercise not only helps you keep trim; it also helps in keeping you fit and strong. Research suggests that people who exercise regularly, 5 times a week, are at a less likely risk of acquiring any kind of heart problem than those who do not exercise. Remaining active means that you have a high dose of HDL or high-density lipoprotein running through your system at all times. This ensures the smooth flow of blood and no fat blockage. Other diseases that are kept at bay because of exercise include diabetes type II, stroke, metabolic syndrome, arthritis, depression and various cancers.

Therefore, if you are on the Ketogenic diet, by no means does it means that you are exempted from the category of people who need to be involved in regular exercise routines. However, there are certain things you will need to keep in mind when working out during the diet.

The first thing to consider is the reason for your diet. Are you following KD to reduce weight or is there some other medical reason involved? Do you suffer from epilepsy, diabetes type II, cancer or Alzheimer's?

If you are following the Ketogenic diet for some medical disease, then you need to consult a doctor before starting any exercise routine. But the exercises mentioned below are risk free and can be followed by most patients. Research suggests that patients who have epilepsy, cancer, diabetes or Alzheimer's have a better chance of staying healthy if they participate in regular exercise.

The key to remaining fit and strong is that you neither under do nor overdo any kind of workout. It is recommended that patients start slow with no more than 10-15 minutes a day and then take it up from there gradually. This is to prevent any reaction or injury that might occur because of sudden physical exertion.

These exercises are light and will not let you feel weak or tired. Instead they will help in developing muscles and keeping you active.

1. **Walking:** A simple and very effective form of aerobic exercise, walking allows you to help with digestion and keeping your muscles strong. It also helps by increasing stamina and range of motion. If you are not used to walking, start by walking for as many minutes as it takes to make you feeling slightly tired. Add a minute every two days and within a week you will be able to walk for 20 minutes without feeling tired.
2. **Biking:** Another cardio exercise, this is particularly beneficial in helping you develop stamina. When you start, do not overdo it. No more than 10-15 minutes for three days and then add 2 more minutes a day for one week.
3. **Crunches:** These are relatively safe and easy. Just make sure that you don't exert yourself or a seizure might occur. Do it at home instead of going to the gym and keep the crunches simple.
4. **Swimming:** Swimming can be great but it must be done under supervision. Even though it is one of the best forms of cardio, swimming can be greatly exerting and sometimes the muscles can become cramped. To avoid this or any seizure, be sure to participate in swimming when someone is with you.
5. **Strength Training:** It is recommended that strength training should also be included after a certain period of exercise. This is because it works to improve the immune system as well as allow the body to grow stronger. But it is highly advised that patients

should never become involved in strength training on their own. They should always seek the help of a professional so that a balance and gradual buildup of resistance can be obtained.

Exercising with KD for Weight Loss

If weight loss is your main goal and you don't have any other health issue, then it is suggested that you work out for 45-60 minutes a day, five days a week to achieve effective weight loss. Aerobic exercise, also known as cardiovascular exercise, is the best that can be followed.

Remember though that the first 2 or 3 weeks your body will need to adjust to the fact that it does not depend on carbohydrates for its energy supply. Research suggests that the body feels relatively weak during this time period, which is why hard-core workout become taxing or difficult. Do not try anything extensive in these first few weeks. Start off by something light like walking or jogging. Once your body becomes attuned to the fuel provided by fats, in about a month, you can increase the intensity of your exercise program.

Many studies show that since the Ketogenic diet can work wonders for those trying to lose weight, the addition of a proper exercise routine means that individuals are able to lose weight faster and then maintain it too. What happens is this; when you exercise while consuming carbs, it takes about 20 minutes for the fats to start burning off. But when you are on the Ketogenic diet, the state of ketosis allows a constant fat burning potential, which means that exercise will encourage an even quicker metabolic rate, helping you lose weight faster.

Another reason why the rate of weight loss increases is that with exercise you develop muscles, which too act as fat burners. Your body shape becomes pronounced and you acquire a lean and toned appearance. The key to this is following a workout program that plays with your strengths. Below are some of the best exercise options for you:

Cardiovascular Workouts

Also known as aerobic exercises, these are those that require a low intensity physical workout routine. The intensity should be such that the heart rate should increase up to

60-85%. Some of the best forms of cardio workout include swimming, long distance running, cycling, dancing and walking. The use of machinery is also very common among cardio practitioners, like treadmill, elliptical machine, stationary bicycle, Stairmaster, indoor rower, etc. Since you want to lose weight through dieting and exercising, it is best you perform 5 days of workout that comprises of different procedures like cardio, lunges, crunches, etc.

Keep in mind though that if you are an avid exerciser, then you might experience the feeling that you aren't able to work out as well as you used to. This is because your body has lost many pounds because of the Ketogenic diet, and finds it difficult to revert back to a high intensity workout routine. Just take it slow and patiently and you will notice a visible change over the weeks as your body gains its strength back.

Using Machines

Another effective workout is with the use of exercising machines. These are basically designed for fitness as well as weight loss options. Below are some of the machines that work best for weight loss. You can either buy one of them or get a membership at the nearest gym and hit the machines for an hour each day!

Treadmill

Treadmills are the best calorie burners. If you don't have the time to go out for a walk or run, then do so at your home or gym. The basic idea is to run on the treadmill until you break out in a sweat. The key to a best workout on a treadmill is not to hold the sidebars for support!

Elliptical Machine

If the treadmill is good, then the elliptical is even better. This is because it is safe for your hips, knees and back, whereas the treadmill might cause some stress and tension on the muscles in those areas. Another benefit is that many elliptical machines have the option of pedaling forward as well as backwards. You can also tone your arms by using the poles that come with the machine.

Rowing Machine

Most people don't have the time to go rowing. No worries, you can simply climb on top of the rowing machine and enjoy the weight loss. This machine works because its system has a water-filled flywheel that produces real resistance for the rower, allowing them to exert and have an elevated heart rate. The best part about this machine is that it works for 80% of your body's muscles.

Stair Stepper or StepMill

This machine has the basic functioning of an escalator, just a much faster one. Considered to be one of the hardest cardio workouts, stair steppers require you to quickly change steps on the moving stairs of the machine. Since exercising on the machine is going against gravity, it exerts extra power thereby allowing you to burn more calories in less time.

This exercise is best for people who have a good balance and have not acquired any foot injury in the past.

Cycling Bike

No time to take out your bike and go for a ride? Well, the cycling bike machine works just as effectively if not better. These bikes can be adjusted to suit the needs of individuals which means that they are relatively more effective than routine bikes and let you burn more calories. Rest assured, their pedals are just as smooth as if you were riding a real bicycle!

Join a Dance Group

One of the best forms of exercise routine is dancing. It is perhaps the most fun and the most effective of cardio programs. It gets your heart rate up, makes you sweat, gets you to stretch and works amazingly well for those who are trying to lose weight! You can choose any dance that you like, do it at home alone or join a group that helps you by motivating and challenging you to go further than your limits. You can even ask your partner, friend or family member to join you in your dancing strategy to lose weight.

Some steps that are particularly beneficial in helping lose weight, making muscles flexible and your bones strong are plié, pulse, staggered wall squat and the salsa workout routine. Not only will you have an amazing time, you will also lose stubborn pounds without noticing how they disappeared!

Take Part in a Physical Fitness Program

There are many physical fitness programs that you can become a part of. Join a gym or go to a group that does stretching exercises on the beach. The thing about joining a workout group is that you end up completing the whole program. You have more motivation, accountability, and people to encourage you with your fitness program and goals.

You can even join an exercise group that is particularly made up of people who are on the Ketogenic diet. This way you will be able to share your diet experiences as well as learn more ways to work out the way which works best.

Yoga

Yoga is a proven meditation routine that has helped many people in achieving weight loss. What yoga does is that it does not only make your body focus physically but also mentally. Your mind and body become attuned to each other, so that when the mind wills something, your body is bound to follow it.

Yoga also helps you in acquiring a toned physique. This is because you position your body in ways that allows for greater flexibility, and being able to stretch your muscles to their maximum potential. This way, if for example, you wish to have a flat stomach, you will be able to get it sooner because yoga poses will speed up the process.

Exercise Routines for Cyclical Ketogenic Diet

Cyclical Ketogenic diet was basically devised for fitness enthusiasts, people who want to lose weight by gaining muscle mass or athletes who want to become physically stronger. Since the primary aim is to become muscular, exercise routines in cyclical Ketogenic diet are more extraneous and vigorous. They require more exertion and can test the limits of your resistance and power. This is the reason why it becomes a must that when you are following the cyclical Ketogenic diet, and have never worked your muscles hard, that you take it slow.

Another factor to keep in mind is the break day. The diet and its routine simply will not be complete without that day, because it is that one day of carbohydrate consumption your muscles or re-storage of glycogen depends on. Always remember that unlike the classic Ketogenic diet which reduces the intake of carbs to a bare minimum, the cyclical Ketogenic diet does require you to have one day where you consume carbs so as to be able to provide your muscles with glycogen, the agent which helps them workout extensively. Without glycogen, you will strain your muscles to the point where the chances of wear and tear increase drastically. So don't ever try to go on the classic Ketogenic diet and work out too hard.

Now that the basics of cyclical Ketogenic diet and how it works are clear, here are some of the exercise routines you can start when on the diet:

Anaerobic Exercise

Anaerobic means the absence of oxygen, hence anaerobic exercises are those that lead to the reduction of oxygen and formation of lactic acid in its presence. Muscles use oxygen for fuel but since that is absent during anaerobic exercises, the muscles rely on glycogen for their energy supplies. Anaerobic reliance only gives short bursts of performance which is why all the exercises span from a few seconds to about 2 minutes.

Some of the reasons why people adopt anaerobic exercise is that they help in developing lean, strong muscles and burn calories more rapidly. It also leads to faster weight loss compared to aerobic or cardiovascular exercises. Anaerobic exercises also help in the development of endurance and resistance. Another advantage of participating in anaerobic exercises is increased capacity for tolerating and excreting lactic acid and thereby being able to fight fatigue better. Some of the best forms of anaerobic exercises include weight lifting and sprinting. If you have never tried anaerobic exercises before, keep the following things in mind:

1. When on the cyclical Ketogenic diet, the first few weeks you will have lower energy levels and will feel relatively weak. This means that it might not be the right time for any exercise, let alone anaerobic exercise. Give yourself at least two to three weeks to settle in to the diet routine and then start exercising gradually.

2. If you aren't used to anaerobic exercise, take things slowly. Start with low intensity aerobic exercise first, develop some fitness and then progress onto anaerobic exercise routines.

3. Before starting any anaerobic exercise, warm up for about 5-10 minutes. This will prepare your body for the upcoming hardcore workout. Once you have completed the workout, cool down for 5-10 minutes.

4. If you have any medical condition, take advice from a medical professional before starting with any anaerobic diet plan. These exercises should also not be taken up by pregnant women.

Below are some of the best forms of anaerobic exercises that you can make a part of your routine:

Heavy Weightlifting

Considered to be the best form of anaerobic exercise, heavy weightlifting requires short bursts of energy and resistance. The key thing is to start lifting weight that is up to your capacity. Start slow and then increase gradually. Evidence that suggests you have the right weight is to be able to maintain a correct posture. Below are some directions for weight lifting:

1. It is always recommended that you never exercise on an empty stomach, but this most certainly does not mean you should start lifting weights the minute after you had dinner. Take a 40 minute break otherwise you will likely experience cramps.

2. Warm up is a must before weight lifting. Your body will get in the routine and will store some oxygen to give your muscles some leverage. One of the easiest warm up sessions is 5 pushups and 5 sit ups, followed by 30 seconds of rest. Then do the same exercises 10 times each with 30 seconds of rest and follow the same process but with 20 of each exercise. Do the procedure backwards once and you have completed your warm up session. This is only one option, you can try anything else that you are comfortable with.

3. Start with the weights that are comfortable yet still require some effort. The best way to check most appropriate weights is to notice that you are not able to do more repetitions than 15-20 times.

4. One of the simplest routines you can follow is start with bench pressing 50 kilos 5 times and a 30 second rest. Then do the same thing 10 times with 30 second rests. Then 15 times and rest. Then 10 times and rest and the last is 5 times. Once you have completed this pyramid, rest for about 1 minute. Do this pyramid three times and then progress onto some cardio exercise.

5. If weight lifting for the first time, start with as many as you can and bring the level up to 30 minutes.

6. Once you have completed the training session, always do a cool down stretch with some simple stretching exercises. The idea is to get your heart beat back to normal pace again.

7. When the stretching is done, go for a hot shower. The water must be hot but not so much that you scald yourself! The hot shower helps in relaxing your muscles and erasing and effects of contraction and fatigue because of the lactic acid buildup.

8. This was only one kind of weight lifting exercise. Make sure you don't just focus on your biceps but other parts of the body too.

9. Once you get used to the weights and lifting them does not seem to be a problem (takes about 8 weeks), increase the number of weights you lift. If you were using say 50 kilos, move on to 70, etc.

Sprinting

Sprints are another form of effective anaerobic exercise. Many people opt for a treadmill, but experts suggest that solid, hard ground is much more beneficial. Sprint is basically a faster version of running. You can start by walking for two minutes and then turning it into a jog for another 3 minutes. Then burst into a sprint for about 1 minutes and 30 seconds. Slow to a jog for 3 minutes and then again repeat the same process. The idea is to get it done for 30 minutes.

When you are new, it will tire you out quickly, so you can start by doing 10 minutes and then taking it up from there.

Bike Sprint

Bike sprinting is similar to running sprints. The difference is that you do it on a bike instead of on foot. A regular bike or stationary bike can be used for the process. The process is the same as running a sprint. All you would need to do is go slow a few minutes and then switch to a mad sprint for 30 seconds to 1 minute. Repeat the same thing for about 30 minutes or build up to 30 minutes.

Swim Sprint

Did you know there is yet another kind of sprint? It is known as the swimming sprint. The process for a swimming sprint is the same as running or bike sprints, with the only difference being that you are in the water. Freestyle of swimming is the best idea with slow swimming for a few minutes followed by sprint swimming for 30 seconds to a 1 or 1 and a half minute.

Out of all the sprints, swimming is perhaps the most difficult because water creates more resistance and you have to make your muscles work harder. This is the reason why it can work even better than the other two.

Punching

This is yet another form of anaerobic exercise. Mostly used by boxers, you can add this to your routine if you like. All you will need is a punching bag and the use of your fists. Simply punch the bag rapidly with the right fist and then the left. Use your hands alternatively and make the progress rapid. You should do it as long as it takes your muscles to become fatigued. Don't overdo it or you may injure some tendon or tissue. Start slow and increase the time duration slowly.

Aerobic Exercise

Cyclical Ketogenic diet is for muscle building but this does not mean you only follow anaerobic exercises. To become fit, the first thing you need to do is start with aerobic exercises to gain enough muscle mass, so as to be able to tolerate hardcore workout routines. Since aerobic exercises require the movement of larger muscles, it ensures that your entire body gets toned and shaped.

Walking, running, swimming, bicycling, dancing and all the cardio mentioned in the Ketogenic exercise section above, are excellent and can be practiced when following the cyclical Ketogenic diet.

When on the cyclical Ketogenic diet, give yourself some time to first get used to the diet. Once your body becomes adapted to the use of fats as fuel providers (it takes about 2-3 weeks), start with easy aerobics, also known as cardio exercises. This will help you in getting your body active and will prepare you for harder and more extensive workout routines.

It takes a month or two before you can switch from aerobic to an anaerobic exercise program. As your body gets used to the workout sessions, you can make the switch. It is recommended that instead of just focusing on any one type of exercise, mix and match the two. For example, you can start with some cardio workout and after 30 minutes switch to anaerobic exercise for another 30 minutes. This will speed up the process of weight loss and will also help you in remaining trim and toned.

Is Cyclical Ketogenic Diet for You?

Cyclical Ketogenic diet, along with a balanced mix of aerobic and anaerobic exercise routines can work wonders for you if you want to lose weight along with building muscles. It takes some time getting used to, but once you have learned the art of using the diet to your advantage, it can be the best tool for you.

The most amazing part about cyclical Ketogenic diet is that it allows you one day of break, where you can eat about anything your heart desires. This means that controlling cravings for food you are otherwise denied becomes a lot easier. You don't have to give up eating; instead you just have to redirect it somewhat. In this diet and exercise, you neither starve nor feel like having eaten less. The feeling of satiety is always achieved. If there is a craving for sugar, you can always satisfy it on the break days!

Just remember that patience and persistence is the key. Also that you need to take the whole experience one day at a time! Neither the diet nor the exercises work over night, but they do show a difference and you start noticing it within the first three months. So if building up your body is your requirement, cyclical Ketogenic diet is the best for you!

How to Tailor it for Yourself

The Ketogenic diet along with proper exercise is one of the best ways to lose weight. This is not just an amateur saying, but decades of scientific research also suggest the same. The great thing about this diet is that it is relatively harmless and does not have any dangerous side effects.

If you are following the Ketogenic diet for weight loss, you don't have to do everything as it says. Of course, the basic diet ratio of 4:2:1 for fats, protein and carbohydrate respectively, has to remain the same, but the rest of it you can modify to suit your individual needs.

Depending on the amount of weight you want to lose, you can diet for some prescribed and pre-determined period only. For example if it's only a few pounds you want to get rid of, then a diet of 3-4 months might be enough for you.

On the other hand, if obesity is the issue, then the Ketogenic diet might need to be followed for some years. Even though the state of ketosis leads you to lose weight quickly, some time is required to make sure that you keep the weight completely off.

Every person has a different level of ketosis. While some can achieve it on 30g of carbs, others can attain it on 70g. This means that you will have to go by trial and error to see what works best for you. Start with the lowest amount of carbohydrates and increase it every day to see whether or not you still get to the state of ketosis. Add the amount of fats and proteins in 4:2 ratio and wait for results.

Even after you are done with the diet, keep in mind that you will have to get rid of all the unhealthy living habits. You will have to adopt a much healthier eating habit and continue with your exercise routine. If you go back to all the previous and unhealthy old ways, then the entire purpose of the diet will be lost and you will revert back to the condition of overweight problems.

When tailoring the diet for yourself, remember that you cannot eat or exercise if you don't like the acts. So make sure that the foods you choose are ones that you enjoy eating and a workout regimen that you have fun with. Otherwise, most people get bored and leave the diet in the middle. One more tip is to not check your weight each day, since weight varies from 2-4 pounds. Instead check your weight every week and note it down so that you remember. Also check your inches every two weeks and note them down too.

How to Lose Weight with Ketogenic Diet in a Week

Weight loss with the Ketogenic diet is not just possible; it is proved by scientific facts. But is it possible to lose weight within a week? The answer is yes. Unbelievable? Not really. Read on to find out more.

What the Ketogenic diet does is eliminate the amount of carbs you consume. From eating say more than 100 grams of carbs a day, you go below 30 grams of carbs a day. And always remember, it is the amount of carbs in a diet which leads to potential weight gain or loss. When you cut down such a huge quantity for a week, it means that you automatically shed the pounds. But how will you get the energy required to keep your body functioning? This fuel comes from fats.

The Ketogenic diet prescribes the use of fats as the 75% of your nutrition supply and the main element in your meal plan of the day. The amount of protein is reduced to 25% and carbohydrates only 5%. This is vastly different from what you are used to eating in your normal routine days.

So what happens is this; you take your body by surprise when you start the Ketogenic diet. Since your body does not expect this reduction in carbohydrate, it is not prepared for any kind of storage. The energy that it used to get from carbs now comes from fats and since fat cannot be reduced and all excess is urinated out, the body is not left with anything to store. What this ultimately means is that you lose about 5-7 pounds in a week. But here's the catch. The weight you lose is mostly water weight which will come right back up as soon as you start eating normally. Is there a solution? Yes there is!

When it is said that you lose weight in the first week, it means the week that comes after the water weight. This may sound like the second week, but in terms of the Ketogenic diet program, it is actually the first week because the weight you lose then is one that can be maintained with care.

Here is how the theory works. When you lose weight seven days after the start of the Ketogenic diet it is 5-7 pounds of the water weight. But the week after, you lose about 4-5 pounds, depending on different people. So after the actual first week of the diet, and not the water weight loss week, you lose up to 8-10 pounds of body weight! Consider how much more weight you will be able to lose if you practiced the diet for 4-6 months!

If you only want to shed 5-6 pounds, then this one week approach to the Ketogenic diet will be ideal for you, as it will help you lose the weight and get in shape. If you also add some light exercise to this routine, the likelihood of losing more weight increases.

If you want to lose more than 5-6 pounds, you can try this diet for a month or two to see the results and take it from there. But whatever you do, your body will lose at least 5-7 pounds the first week because of drastic dietary changes!

Food List Based on the Ketogenic Diet

Below is a list of foods that are allowed and recommended during the Ketogenic diet. Make sure you do not eat anything that is sugary or has a high amounts of carbs. The list below contains foods that are easily available at all markets and stores.

Meat

1. Chicken
2. Bacon, ham, sausage
3. Beef roast
4. All kinds of seafood *except lobsters and clams*
5. Shellfish
6. Lamb
7. Goat
8. Veal
9. Pork
10. Turkey, quail, goose, pheasant, duck

Dairy Products

1. Eggs
2. Creams *except heavy, sour, whipped*
3. Butter
4. Cheese
5. Yogurt
6. Milk *in moderation*

Vegetables

1. Broccoli
2. Asparagus
3. Cucumbers
4. Olives

5. Lettuce
6. Artichoke hearts
7. Green bell peppers
8. Any green leafy vegetable
9. Brussels sprouts
10. Celery
11. Kale
12. Mushrooms
13. Shallots
14. Spinach
15. Snow peas
16. Turnips
17. Leeks
18. Bok Choy
19. Cauliflower
20. Garlic

Fruits

1. Avocados
2. Berries *in restricted amounts*

Most fruits have high sugar content, so avoid them while on the diet. If you must have something, keep the carbs intake in mind.

Nuts and Seeds

1. Macadamia
2. Almonds
3. Hazelnuts
4. Pecans
5. Walnuts
6. Sunflower seeds
7. Pumpkin seeds

8. Sesame seeds

Make sure you consume them in limited amounts because they can be high in carbs.

Spices

1. Basil
2. Black pepper
3. Cayenne pepper
4. Chili pepper
5. Cilantro seeds
6. Peppermint
7. Sage
8. Thyme
9. Turmeric
10. Cloves

Remember that most spices have high carbs content so consume them in lesser quantities.

Miscellaneous

These are the foods you can eat, but be sure to keep an eye out for how much you consume.

1. Mustard
2. Mayonnaise
3. Ketchup
4. Soy sauce
5. Decaf tea and coffee
6. Salsa
7. Almond flour or other nut flour
8. Lemon or lime juice (1 gram of carb per tablespoon)
9. Vinegar *less quantity*
10. Sugar-free salad dressings

11. Unsweetened cocoa powder

12. Dark chocolate *in restricted amounts*

Foods to Avoid

1. Bread of all kinds

2. Sugars of all kinds

3. Rice, pasta, wheat

4. Beans and lentils

5. Potatoes, carrots, corn, okra and tomatoes

6. Almost all the fruits

7. Soft drinks and soda

8. Processed and preserved foods

All the above mentioned foods contain high amounts of sugar, so forget about them while you are on the Ketogenic diet.

30 Recipes for the Ketogenic Diet

This section of the eBook contains 30 delicious recipes based on the theory of the Ketogenic diet. You can change certain ingredients but make sure that the ones you replace are not rich in carbohydrates.

Breakfast

Breakfast is the start of the day and needs to be healthy and satisfying. These 5 recipes given below will make you full and give you energy. Have fun cooking them!

1. Keto Eggs Frijoles

Serving Size

Serves 4

Preparation Time & Cooking Time

Prep time: 10 minutes

Cooking Time: 20 minutes

Ingredients

Chopped onion, ½

Lightly beaten eggs, 4

Fresh salsa, 1 cup

Minced garlic, 2 cloves

Cayenne pepper, 1/3 tsp

Lettuce leaves, 4

Pinto beans, ½ cup

Butter, 3 tsp

Sea salt, a pinch

Process

Heat up 2 tsp butter in a nonstick pan and cook onions, garlic and sea salt for about 7 minutes. Then add beans and cayenne pepper and cook on low heat for 12 minutes. Cover with lid and set aside.

In another pan, heat 1 tsp butter and cook eggs in a scrambled eggs style for 4 minutes. Keep aside. Take leaves of lettuce and spread them in a dish. First put bean mixture, top with eggs and salsa. Serve immediately.

Nutritional Info

Calories: 230.9

Fats: 12.5g

Proteins: 9.3g

Carbs: 18.6g

Serving Size

Serves 6

Preparation Time & Cooking Time

Prep time: 10 minutes

Cooking time: 60 minutes

Ingredients

Almond flour, 1 ¼ cup

Baking powder, 1 tsp

Egg whites, 4

Apple cider vinegar, 2 tbsp

Psyllium husk powder, 1 tbsp

Boiling water, 1 cup

Sea salt, a pinch

Process

Preheat oven at 350 degrees F. Mix all the ingredients together except water. Then using a hand mixer, add in water a little at a time. Mix well and separate into 6 equal sized buns. Place them in a parchment lined baking tray and bake for 60 minutes. Let cool and then cut them and use as you like.

Nutritional Info

Calories: 167

Fats: 12g

Protein: 5 g

Carbs: 7g

3. Coffee Smoothie

Serving Size

Serves 1

Preparation Time & Cooking Time

Prep time: 5 minutes

Cooking time: 0

Ingredients

Espresso, 1 shot

Cinnamon, a pinch

Yogurt, ¼ cup

Stevia, a pinch

Ice cubes, as required

Process

Combine all the ingredients in the blender and process until smooth. Drink the delicious coffee smoothie immediately.

Nutritional Info

Calories: 169

Fats: 2g

Proteins: 35g

Carbs: 3g

4. Egg Omelet

Serving Size

Serves 1

Preparation Time & Cooking Time

Prep time: 5 minutes

Cooking time: 6 minutes

Ingredients

Egg whites, 4

Egg yolk, 1

Shredded spinach, ½ cup

Chopped onion, 1 tbsp

Almond milk, 2 tbsp

Basil, 1 pinch

Olive oil, 2 tbsp

Sea salt, a pinch

Process

Beat egg whites and yolk and add almond milk to it and set aside. In a pan add olive oil and sauté spinach and onion. When the veggies turn soft, then add egg mixture to it. Let the eggs stiffen a little and then turn. Fry until golden on both sides. Serve warm.

Nutritional Info

Calories: 203

Fats: 5g

Proteins: 20g

Carbs: 10g

Serving Size

Serves 1

Preparation Time & Cooking Time

Prep time: 3 minutes

Cooking time: 20 minutes

Ingredients

Egg, 1

Coconut flour, 1 tsp

Mozzarella cheese, ¾ cup

Cream cheese, 2 tbsp

Olive oil, 1 tbsp

Dried Italian herbs, ½ tsp

Sea salt and pepper, to taste

Process

Preheat oven to 350 degrees F. Make sure that both the cheeses are at room temperature. Beat egg and add all other ingredients to it, mixing well. On a lined baking sheet, spread the mixture in such a way that it makes a circular shape of about 8 inches. Bake for 18-20 minutes in the center of the oven. Turn the bread 5 minutes before taking it out of the oven. This way, both sides will be crisp.

Nutritional Info

Calories: 479

Fats: 4g

Proteins: 27g

Carbs: 3.9g

Serving Size

Yields 3 cups

Preparation Time & Cooking Time

Prep time: 5 minutes

Cooking time: 10 minutes

Ingredients

Eggs, 12

Mayonnaise, ½ cup

Minced onion, 1/3 cup

Butter, 2 tbsp

Mustard, ½ tsp

Sea salt and pepper, 1 tsp

Process

Fill a pot with cold water and place all the eggs in it. Bring the water to a boil and then cook for another 10 minutes. Take the pan off heat and strain out all the water. Fill the pot with cold water again and let the eggs sit in it for 2 to 3 minutes. Then take out the eggs, peel off their shells and chop them. Add in the rest of the ingredients and serve with rolls or Keto bread.

Nutritional Info

Calories: 163

Fats: 14g

Proteins: 6g

Carbs: 2g

Lunch

These yummy lunch recipes will definitely leave you asking for more. Just make sure you eat well but do not overeat!

Serving Size

Serves 12

Preparation Time & Cooking Time

Prep time: 20 minutes

Cooking time: 30 minutes

Ingredients

Eggs, 12

Finely chopped onion, 1

Heavy cream, 2 cups

Shredded Colby jack cheese, 5 cups (divide into two parts)

Chopped cauliflower, ½ cup

Butter, 3 tbsp

Bacon, 12 slices

Thyme, 2 tsp

Sea salt and pepper, 1 tsp

Process

Preheat oven to 350 degrees F. Heat 2 tbsp butter on medium low-heat and sauté onions and cauliflower until soft. Set aside for later use.

Take raw bacon slices and spread them on a lined baking tray, and bake them for 20 minutes. When they are done, let them cool and then crumble into small pieces. In a bowl, beat eggs and add cream and spices. Mix well. Then add bacon pieces and whisk until well combined.

Take two inch pans and butter them with the remaining butter. Take the Colby cheese and lay two cups in the bottom of each pan. Then add ½ of the veggies and ½ of the cream, eggs and bacon mixture. Make sure the mixture is spread evenly.

Put the quiche in the oven and bake for 25-28 minutes. Check with a knife inserted in the middle to see if it's done. Serve hot.

Nutritional Info

Each slice has,

Calories: 382

Fats: 33g

Proteins: 16g

Carbs: 6g

Serving Size

Serves 10-15

Preparation Time & Cooking Time

Prep time: 10-12 minutes

Cooking time: 20-25 minutes

Ingredients

Minced onions, 4 ounces

Cold ricotta cheese, 1 cup

Ground beef, 1 pound

Hard dry cheese of your choice, 4 ounces

Large cold whole egg, 1

Butter, 2 tbsp

Herb seasoning, 3 tsp

Pepper, 1 tsp

Sea salt, 1 tsp

Process

Preheat oven to 350 degrees F. Heat butter in a pan and sauté onions until tender. Let cool completely. Put the hard cheese in the food processor and pulse until it gets crumbly.

In a bowl, combine ricotta cheese and egg, whisk well. Then add the herb seasoning, salt and pepper and mix well. Pour in the crumbly cheese and onions and combine well. Then add the beef and mix again.

Separate the mixture in such a way that you are able to make 1 ounce balls. The end result should be about 30-32 balls. Place them on a lined baking sheet and bake for 20 minutes or until cooked through.

Nutritional Info

One meatball contains,

Calories: 75

Fats: 5g

Proteins: 6g

Carbs: 1g

9. Baked Salmon

Serving Size

Serves 1-2

Preparation Time & Cooking Time

Prep time: 1 hour

Cooking time: 20-30 minutes

Ingredients

Salmon fillets, 2 pounds (sliced into ½ pound pieces)

Chopped mushrooms, ½ cup

Chopped green onions, ½ cup

Minced garlic, 1 tsp

Ground ginger, ½ tsp

Butter, 4 ounces

Sesame oil, 4 ounces

Tamari soy sauce, ½ cup

Basil, ½ tsp

Oregano leaves, 1 tsp

Thyme, ¼ tsp

Rosemary, ½ tsp

Tarragon, ¼ tsp

Process

Mix sesame oil, all spices and tamari soy sauce together and pour into a large Ziploc bag. Add the salmon fillets and shake a little. Refrigerate for about 1 hour or more to marinate.

Preheat oven to 350 degrees F. Take out the fish from the fridge and put it, along with marinade into a lined baking tray. Bake for 10-15 minutes.

Heat butter in a pan and add veggies to it. Sauté for 3-5 minutes. Take off heat and pour this mixture over fillets, covering them well with butter. Put back in oven and bake for another 10 minutes. Serve immediately.

Nutritional Info

Calories: 353

Fats: 23g

Proteins: 32g

Carbs: 2g

Serving Size

Serves 2-3

Preparation Time & Cooking Time

Prep time: 10 minutes

Cooking time: About 1 hour

Ingredients

Shredded raw green cabbage, 30g

Chicken broth, 100g

Diced garlic, 1g

Diced cooked chicken breast, 20g

Diced onion, 5g

Olive oil, 15g

Butter, 15g

Mayonnaise, 15g

Sea salt and pepper, to taste

Process

Mix butter and olive oil and heat in a pan over medium-low heat. Put cabbage, garlic and onion into this mixture and cook until veggies start softening. Then add chicken and broth into the vegetables, cover and let simmer over low heat. When the vegetables become completely soft, remove from heat and mix in mayo. Then pour the mixture into a blender and process until smooth. Serve immediately.

You can also serve this with flat bread or Keto rolls.

Nutritional Info

Calories: 397

Fats: 9g

Proteins: 7.3g

Carbs: 2.5g

11. Stir Fry Beef

Serving Size

Serves 3

Preparation Time & Cooking Time

Prep time: 8 minutes

Cooking time: 15 minutes

Ingredients

Kale leaves, 2

Broccoli, ½ cup

Spanish onion, ½

Brown mushrooms, 5

Ground beef, 300g

Cayenne pepper, 1 tbsp

Red pepper, ½

Chinese five spices. 1 tbsp

Coconut oil, 1 tbsp

Process

Chop all the veggies and cook in heated oil until soft. Then add in ground beef, as well as the spices and cook for 3 minutes. Cover the pan and cook for another 10 minutes or until beef is brown. Serve hot.

Nutritional Info

Calories: 307

Fats: 18g

Proteins: 29g

Carbs: 7g

12.   Cheesy Salami Cannoli

Serving Size

Yields 5 cannoli

Preparation Time & Cooking Time

Prep time: 10 minutes

Cooking time: -

Ingredients

Cream cheese, 2 ounce

Thinly sliced salami, 10 slices

Chopped green onion, 1 tbsp

Cayenne pepper, ½ tsp

Sea salt, to taste

Process

Mix together cream cheese, green onion, salt and cayenne. Then put one slice of salami on top of another and spread it with the cream mixture. Roll the salami in a cannoli shape and serve.

Nutritional Info

Calories: 193

Fats: 17g

Proteins: 8g

Carbs: 2g

Dinner

Below are some of the most filling and mouthwatering dinner recipes. Just make sure you eat before 7 o'clock and do not go to bed immediately after eating!

13. Keto Casserole

Serving Size

Serves 5-7

Preparation Time & Cooking Time

Prep time: 20 minutes

Cooking time: 20 minutes

Ingredients

Diced corned beef, ½ pound

Cream cheese, 8 ounce

Sauerkraut, 1 can (drained)

Shredded Swiss cheese, 2 cups

Pickle brine, 2 tbsp

Mayonnaise, ½ cup

Caraway seeds, ½ tsp

Vinegar, 1 tsp

Salt and garlic salt, a pinch

Process

Preheat oven to 350 degrees F. Melt cream cheese in a pan on low heat and add mayo to it. Cut your corned beef in half inch slices and add this along with 1 ½ cups of Swiss cheese and sauerkraut into the simmering cream cheese. Mix well and take off the heat. Season it with salt, vinegar and garlic salt.

Pour this mixture in a greased baking dish and sprinkle leftover cheese and seeds on top. Bake for about 20 minutes or until the top of the mixture starts bubbling.

Nutritional Info

Calories: 360

Fats: 25g

Proteins: 14g

Carbs: 5g

Serving Size

Serves 1

Preparation Time & Cooking Time

Prep time: 8 minutes

Cooking time: 15 minutes

Ingredients

Portobello mushroom caps, 2

Garlic clove, 1

Olive oil, ½ tbsp

Sea salt and pepper, to taste

Grass-fed ground beef, 6 ounce

Cheddar cheese, ¼ cup

Sea salt and pepper, to taste

Dijon mustard, 1 tbsp

Process

Preheat griddle to high. In a bowl, mix together olive oil, salt, garlic and pepper and put the Portobello mushroom caps in this to marinate.

In another bowl, mix ground beef, salt, cheese, mustard and pepper together. Form into 2 inch patties.

Put your mushroom caps on the grill for about 8 minutes to cook. Put the burger patties on the grill for 5 minutes. When they are both done, take them off on a plate, put burger patties in between the two mushroom caps (these act as buns), pour on some ketchup and enjoy!

Nutritional Info

Calories: 735

Fats: 48g

Proteins: 60g

Carbs: 8g

Serving Size

Yields 10 chicken pieces

Preparation Time & Cooking Time

Prep time: 10 minutes

Cooking time: 30 minutes

Ingredients

Plain whey protein, ¾ cup

Crushed pork rinds, 1 cup

Boneless chicken pieces, 10 (breast, leg or wings)

Heavy cream, ¼ cup

Eggs, 2

Parmesan cheese, ½ cup

Seafood spice blend, 1 tsp

Onion powder, ½ tsp

Sea salt and pepper, to taste

Water, ¼ cup

Palm shortening, 1 ¼ cup

Process

Put all the dry ingredients in a paper bag and shake well. Whisk together eggs, cream and water in a bowl and set aside. First dip your chicken pieces in the wet mixture and then put your chicken pieces, 3 at a time in the paper bag and shake well to coat. Fry them in the hot palm shortening. Cook for as long as it takes both the sides to turn brown and crispy. Take out on a paper towel and serve hot!

Nutritional Info

For one chicken piece,

Calories: 113.4

Fats: 7.26g

Proteins: 12.8g

Carbs: 1.72g

16. Keto Tuscan Soup

Serving Size

Serves 8

Preparation Time & Cooking Time

Prep time: 20 minutes

Cooking time: 45 minutes

Ingredients

Chicken stock, 2 cups

Ground Italian sausage, 1 pound

Chopped kale, 3 cups

Diced cauliflower, 2 cups

Water, 1 quart

Butter, ¼ cup and 1 tbsp

Chopped garlic, 2 cloves

Crushed red pepper 1 tbsp

Sea salt and pepper, to taste

Heavy whipping cream, 2 tbsp

Process

Heat up 1 tbsp butter in a pan and sauté garlic. Add sausage and cook until they turn brown. Once it's done, add chicken stock, water, salt, crushed red pepper and black pepper. Cook on low heat for half an hour. Then add kale, cauliflower and the rest of the butter, cooking for 15-20 minutes or as long as it takes for the veggies to become soft. Before serving, add the whipping cream.

Nutritional Info

Calories: 243

Fats: 21g

Proteins: 9g

Carbs: 4g

Serving Size

Serves 2

Preparation Time & Cooking Time

Prep Time: 2 hour

Cooking time: 6 minutes

Ingredients

Boneless pork chops, 4

Halved garlic cloves, 4

Almond flour, 1 tbsp

Medium star anise, 1

Peeled and diced stalk lemongrass, 1

Fish sauce, 1 tbsp

Sesame oil, 1 tsp

Peppercorns, 1.2 tsp

Ketchup, ½ tbsp

Sambal chili paste, ½ tbsp

Five spice, ½ tsp

Soy sauce, 1 ½ tsp

Process

Put your pork chops on a flat surface and beat them with a rolling pin, until they get flattened to the thickness of ½ inch. In a blender, grind star anise and peppercorn so that it turns into powder. Add garlic and lemon grass and blend until it all turns into a paste. Add soy sauce, fish sauce, five spice and sesame oil and mix well. This is your marinade. Coat the pork chops with this on both sides and leave at room temperature for about an hour.

Then coat the chops with almond flour and fry in a heated pan for 2 minutes on each side. When a golden brown crust is formed, remove from heat. Cut pork chop in strips and serve on a platter.

Mix together Sambal chili paste and ketchup and spread this sauce over the pork chops. Serve immediately.

Nutritional Info

Calories: 544

Fats: 19g

Proteins: 68g

Carbs: 12g

Serving Size

Serves 4

Preparation Time & Cooking Time

Prep time: 10-15 minutes

Cooking time: About 1 hour

Ingredients

Chicken thighs, 3 pounds

Heavy whipping cream, ½ cup

Chopped cheese, 7 ounce

Crushed tomatoes, 1 cup

Water, 1 cup

Butter, 4 tbsp

Garlic and ginger paste, 3 tbsp

Cilantro, 5 springs

Olive oil, 1 tbsp

Coconut oil, 2 tsp

Garam masala, 1 tsp

Paprika, 1.2 tsp

Red chili powder, ½ tsp

Coriander powder, 1 tsp

Sea salt, 1 tsp

Pepper, 1 tsp

Process

Preheat oven to 375 degrees F. Mix olive oil and salt and rub it on chicken. Then put it in a lined baking tray and let bake for 25 minutes. In a pan, heat up butter and coconut oil. Then add ginger, garlic paste and cook for 2 minutes. Add tomatoes, Garam masala, red chili powder, coriander powder, paprika, salt and pepper. Cook until the oil comes on top. Add in the cheese and water and let cook on a low flame for about 5 minutes. Then add in cream and mix well.

Meanwhile, take out the cooked chicken from the oven and remove bones. When the curry starts boiling add in the chicken pieces. Mix and let cook for another 5 minutes. Add cilantro on top and serve hot!

Nutritional Info

Calories: 1956

Fats: 175g

Proteins: 69g

Carbs: 20g

Desserts

These yummy deserts will have you licking your fingers! But try not to eat too much or your diet will be ruined!

19. Coconut and Cream Macaroons

Serving Size

Yields 56

Preparation Time & Cooking Time

Prep time: 40 minutes

Cooking time: 25 minutes

Ingredients

Softened cream cheese, 8 ounces

Heavy cream, 2 ounces

Finely shredded dried coconut, 16 ounces (unsweetened)

Egg whites, 4

Erythritol, 1 cup

Cream of tartar, ¼ tsp

Vanilla, 1 tsp

Unsweetened white chocolate syrup, 2 ounces

Dark chocolate chips, 2 ounces

Process

Preheat oven to 325 degrees F. In a bowl, combine egg whites, cream of tartar and vanilla and beat with an electric mixer on high speed for as long as it takes to form soft peaks. Then add erythritol 1 tbsp at a time, beating all the while so that the soft peaks turn stiff. Then fold coconut in the mixture.

In a separate bowl, beat cream cheese and heavy cream until smooth. Pour syrup in and combine well. Then mix coconut mixture into the cream mixture stirring gently. Add in the chocolate chips and mix well.

On a parchment paper lined cookie sheet, pour 1 inch scoops and place in the oven. Bake for 25 minutes and then turn off the heat. Let the macaroons stay in the oven for another 30 minutes. Then take out and let cool. Serve.

Nutritional Info

For 1 macaroon,

Calories: 78

Fats: 7g

Proteins: 2g

Carbs: 3g

20. Chocolaty Caramel Muffins

Serving Size

Yields 45 muffins

Preparation Time & Cooking Time

Prep time: 15 minutes

Cooking time: 25 minutes

Ingredients

Unsweetened cooking chocolate, ½ cup

Caramel dip, 1/3 cup

Almond flour, 2 cups

Large eggs, 2

Sour cream, 1 cup

Butter, 2 tbsp

Baking soda, ½ tsp

Erythritol, 1/8 cup

Xanthan gum, ½ tsp

Stevia glycerite, 1 tsp

Process

Preheat oven to 350 degrees F. Whisk together flour, baking soda, xanthan gum and erythritol and set aside. In another bowl, beat eggs and add sour cream, butter, melted cooking chocolate, caramel dip and stevia to it. Add the wet ingredients to the dry and mix well. Pour this batter into a lined cupcake tray, filling about ¾ of each cup. Bake for 25 minutes or until golden. Take out and let cool, then remove the paper liners.

Nutritional Info

Calories: 63

Fats: 5g

Proteins: 2g

Carbs: 3g

Serving Size

Yields 56 cookies

Preparation Time & Cooking Time

Prep time: 15 minutes

Cooking time: 12 minutes

Ingredients

Large eggs, 2

Butter, 2 tbsp

Almond flour, 2 cups

Softened cream cheese, 4 ounces

Powdered erythritol, 2/3 cup

Natural peanut butter, 1 cup (unsweetened)

Honey, ½ cup

Stevia glycerite, 1 tsp

Vanilla extract, 2 tsp

Xanthan gum, 1/8 tsp

Baking soda, 1 tsp

EZSweet liquid splenda, 5 drops

Process

Preheat oven to 350 degrees F. Whisk together flour, baking soda and xanthan gum. Set aside for later use. In another bowl, mix together butter, cream cheese and peanut butter. Use an electric blender on high until the mixture turns smooth. Add honey and sweeteners and keep beating until it turns soft and fluffy. Add in vanilla extract and one egg at a time, beating all the while. Then fold in flour mixture. Combine well. The mixture should now look like shiny dough.

Take a tablespoon and scoop out a spoonful, putting them in your hand. Roll balls and put on a lined baking tray. Press lightly so that it looks like a thick biscuit. Bake for about 12 minutes.

Nutritional Info

For 1 cookie,

Calories: 57

Fats: 5g

Proteins: 3g

Carbs: 3g

Serving Size

Serves 3

Preparation Time & Cooking Time

Prep time: 5 minutes

Cooking time: -

Ingredients

Heavy whipping cream, 4 ounces

Softened cream cheese, 8 ounces

Melted cooking chocolate, 1 ounce (dark chocolate)

Liquid stevia, 5 drops

Process

Mix all the ingredients together and portion out into three bowls. Chill until set and serve immediately. You can top it with a dollop of whipped cream.

Nutritional Info

For 1 serving,

Calories: 424

Fats: 43g

Proteins: 7g

Carbs: 4g

23. Quick Cheesecake

Serving Size

Serves 1

Preparation Time & Cooking Time

Prep time: 5 minutes

Cooking time: 1 ½ minute

Ingredients

Softened cream cheese, 2 ounces

Egg, 1

Powdered erythritol, 2 tbsp

Stevia, 2 tbsp

Heavy cream, 2 tbsp

Lemon juice, ½ tsp

Vanilla, ¼ tsp

Process

Mix all the ingredients in a bowl and whisk until well combined. Pour in a mug and place in the microwave for 1 ½ minutes. Take out after every 30 seconds and mix. When done, refrigerate until set. Top with some blueberries and serve.

Nutritional Info

Calories: 300

Fats: 27.6g

Proteins: 11g

Carbs: 2.5g

Serving Size

Yields 6

Preparation Time & Cooking Time

Prep time: 2 hours

Cooking time: 5 minutes

Ingredients

Cocoa powder, 2 tbsp

Fresh raspberry syrup, 2 tbsp

Butter, 5 tbsp

Coconut oil, 3 tbsp

Process

Put all the ingredients in a pan and cook over low heat. As soon as the mixture turns smooth, pour into some twisty shaped molds and put in the freezer for 2-4 hours. When set, take out and consume immediately. If left at room temperature for too long, they will melt.

Nutritional Info

Calories: 100

Fats: 10g

Proteins: 1g

Carbs: 1g

Snacks

These snacks are ideal for when you feel hungry but it's not time for either lunch or dinner. Try to eat only a little bit or you might ruin your appetite!

25. Garlicky Cheddar Biscuits

Serving Size

Yields 37 biscuits

Preparation Time & Cooking Time

Prep time: 10 minutes

Cooking time: 25 minutes

Ingredients

Large eggs, 2

Cream cheese, 8 ounces

Shredded Colby cheese, 6 ounces

Almond flour, 2 ½ cups

Butter, 5 tbsp

Garlic, 2 tsp

Xanthan gum, 3/2 tsp

Baking soda, 1 tsp

Sea salt, 1 tsp

Process

Preheat oven to 325 degrees F. Put 1 cup almond flour and Colby cheese in the food processor and pulse until fine. Then in a glass bowl, pour cream cheese and butter and microwave for 30 seconds. Whisk until well combined and then add in eggs. Mix in garlic, xanthan gum, baking soda and salt. Add in the almond flour mixture and combine well.

Using a tablespoon, pour a spoonful of the mixture at a time on a lined baking tray. Bake for 25 minutes or until golden brown. Take out and let cool.

Nutritional Info

1 biscuit contains,

Calories: 97

Fats: 35g

Proteins: 3g

Carbs: 9g

26. Tiny Cheesy Muffins

Serving Size

Yields 12 muffins

Preparation Time & Cooking Time

Prep time: 8 minutes

Cooking time: 20 minutes

Ingredients

Egg, 1

Almond flour, 1 cup

Shredded Colby jack cheese, ¼ cup

Minced shallots, ¼ cup

Melted butter, 3 tbsp

Sour cream, 3 tbsp

Sea salt, ½ tsp

Process

Preheat oven to 350 degrees F. Combine wet and dry ingredients separately and then pour the wet into the dry ingredients. Mix well. Scoop the mixture into lined paper liners of the muffin tray and bake for 20 minutes. Take out and let cool for an hour or so. Serve.

Nutritional Info

1 muffin has,

Calories: 97

Fats: 9g

Proteins: 3g

Carbs: 3g

27. Keto Mayo

Serving Size

Yields 1 cup

Preparation Time & Cooking Time

Prep time: 5 minute

Cooking time: -

Ingredients

Egg, 1

Egg yolk, 1

Olive oil, 1 cup

Apple cider vinegar, 2 tsp

Mustard powder, ½ tsp

Lemon juice, 1 tsp

Stevia, A pinch

Sea salt, ½ tsp

Process

Pour all ingredients, except oil, in a bowl. Combine using a hand blender and mix well. Then start adding oil slowly, blending all the time. Keep blending until the mixture thickens and takes the consistency of cream. This mayo can be used with any food you like, or simply gobble it up with crackers!

<u>Nutritional Info</u>

Per 1 tablespoon,

Calories: 113

Fats: 12.73g

Proteins: 0.57g

Carbs: 0.14g

28. Jicama Chipotle Hash

Serving Size

Serves 2

Preparation Time & Cooking Time

Prep time: 2 minutes

Cooking time: 10 minutes

Ingredients

Peeled and diced jicama, 12 ounces

Chopped onion, 4 ounces

Seeded and chopped green bell pepper, 1 ounces

Chopped bacon, 4

Chipotle mayo, 4 tbsp

Process

Put bacon in a pan and cook until brown. Take out on a paper towel to drain and set aside. In the same pan, cook jicama and onions until brown. Then add bell peppers and cook until tender. Take out in a plate.

For the chipotle mayo, simply add 1 tsp of smoky chipotle spice blend in 4 tbsp of mayo. Pour this mayo over the hash and enjoy!

Nutritional Info

Calories: 547

Fats: 48g

Proteins: 14.3g

Carbs: 21.15g

29. Crackers

Serving Size

Yields 30 crackers

Preparation Time & Cooking Time

Prep time: 10 minutes

Cooking time: 20 minutes

Ingredients

Almond flour, 1 ¼ cups

Sour cream, 2 tbsp

Shredded cheddar cheese, ½ cup

Shredded parmesan cheese, ¼ cup

Egg, 1

Melted butter, 2 tbsp

Baking soda, ¼ tsp

Sea salt, to taste

Process

Preheat oven to 350 degrees F. In a bowl combine all the dry ingredients and set aside for later use. Wisk all the wet ingredients together and then pour them into the dry ingredients. Combine well so that a soft dough is formed.

Lay a parchment sheet on a flat surface and put dough on top. Place another parchment sheet on top and roll the dough out in an even thickness. Remove the parchment paper and cut the dough into 2 inch squares.

Put the squares on a lined baking tray and bake for 20 minutes. Let cool for an hour before serving.

Nutritional Info

Calories: 45

Fats: 4g

Proteins: 2g

Carbs: 1g

Serving Size

Yields 12 ounces

Preparation Time & Cooking Time

Prep time: 10 minutes

Cooking time: 50 seconds

Ingredients

Mayonnaise, 2 ounces

Canned pink salmon, 4.35 ounces

Steamed shrimp, 3 ounces

Dried dill, ½ tsp

Cream cheese, 4.5 ounces

Lemon juice, 1 tsp

Sea salt and pepper, to taste

Process

Place cream cheese in a glass bowl and microwave for 50 seconds so that it melts. Add in mayo, lemon juice and spices. Mix well. Put fish and shrimp in a food processor and pulse for 10 seconds. Add in mayo mixture and process for another 40 seconds. Take out in a bowl and serve.

Nutritional Info

Calories: 1136

Fats: 98g

Proteins: 56g

Carbs: 7.2g

Conclusion

And here you have it, everything that you need to know about the Ketogenic diet. The diet is about as safe as can be, but it is still advised to consult with a medical professional before starting it. You can change a few things here and there to suit your requirements just remember maintaining the ratio is the key to success. Best of luck with attaining your weight loss goals!

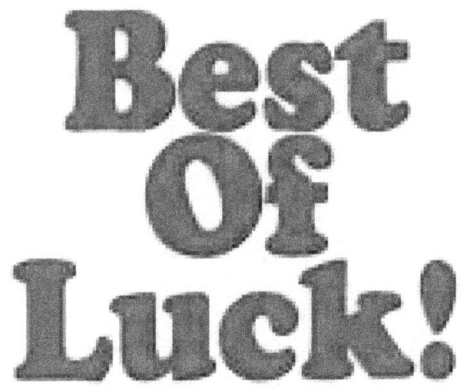